THE ZERO POINT AIR FRYER COOKBOOK 2025

DR. SUSAN COWELL

Copyright © 2024 by Dr. Susan Cowell

All rights reserved. No part of this publication may be reproduced, distributed, or transmitted in any form or by any means, including photocopying, recording, or other electronic or mechanical methods, without the prior written permission of the publisher, except in the case of brief quotations embodied in critical reviews and certain other noncommercial uses permitted by copyright law.

Disclaimer

This book is intended for informational purposes only and is not a substitute for professional medical advice, diagnosis, or treatment. Always consult with a healthcare provider before making significant changes to your diet or lifestyle. The authors and publishers are not liable for any adverse effects resulting from the use or misuse of the information presented herein.

TABLE OF CONTENT

Introduction to The Zero Point Air Fryer Cookbook 9
    What You'll Learn 10
    Who Is This Book For? 12
    Get Ready to Transform Your Kitchen 12
    What Exactly is Zero Point Air Fryer Recipes 13
    Benefits of Zero-Point Air Fryer Recipes 15
    How to Use an Air Fryer with Benefits 15
    Benefits of Using an Air Fryer 17
    Pro Tips for Air Fryer Success 18

CHAPTER ONE 23
    Zero Point Meal Planning: A Guide to Healthy, Guilt-Free Eating
.... 23
    Benefits of Zero Point Meal Planning 24
    How to Start a Zero Point Meal Plan 25
    Pro Tips for Zero Point Meal Planning 27
    Why Zero Point Meal Planning Works 28

CHAPTER ONE 29
    14 Day Zero Point Air Fryer Meal Planning Recipes 29
    Day 1 29

Day 2 30

Day 3 30

Day 4 31

Day 5 32

Day 6 33

Day 7 33

Day 8 34

Day 9 35

Day 10 35

Day 11 36

Day 12 37

Day 13 38

Day 14 38

CHAPTER TWO 41

Zero Point Air Fryer Breakfast Recipes 41

1. Air-Fried Veggie Egg Cups 41

2. Air-Fried Sweet Potato Hash 42

3. Air-Fried Banana Pancakes (Zero Point Style) 43

4. Air-Fried Apple Cinnamon Chips 44

5. Air-Fried Breakfast Quesadilla 44

6. Air-Fried Avocado Toast (Zero Point Style) 45

7. Air-Fried Apple Cinnamon Oats.. 46

8. Air-Fried Veggie Frittata Bites 47

9. Air-Fried Breakfast Stuffed Peppers..................................... 48

10. Air-Fried Zucchini Boats with Eggs................................... 49

11. Air-Fried Breakfast Veggie Quesadilla 50

12. Air-Fried French Toast Sticks (Zero Point Style)............... 51

13. Air-Fried Sweet Potato Breakfast Bites.............................. 52

14. Air-Fried Mini Breakfast Frittatas 52

15. Air-Fried Oatmeal Cups with Berries 53

CHAPTER THREE 55

Zero Point Air Fryer Lunch Recipes.. 55

1. Air-Fried Veggie Fajitas 55

2. Air-Fried Chickpea Salad Wrap.. 56

3. Air-Fried Cauliflower Steaks 57

4. Air-Fried Veggie Burgers 58

5. Air-Fried Stuffed Bell Peppers 59

6. Air-Fried Veggie Tacos 60

7. Air-Fried Falafel 61

8. Air-Fried Sweet Potato Fries 62

9. Air-Fried Portobello Mushroom Burgers 63

10. Air-Fried Eggplant Parmesan 64

11. Air-Fried Stuffed Zucchini Boats 65

12. Air-Fried Veggie-Stuffed Mushrooms 66

13. Air-Fried Spicy Tofu Bites 67

14. Air-Fried Avocado Toast 67

15. Air-Fried Veggie & Bean Wrap 68

CHAPTER FOUR 71

Zero Point Air Fryer Dinner Recipes 71

1. Air-Fried Lemon Garlic Shrimp with Zoodles 71

2. Air-Fried Turkey Meatballs with Marinara Sauce 72

3. Air-Fried Herb-Crusted Salmon 73

4. Air-Fried Chicken and Veggie Skewers 74

5. Air-Fried Eggplant Lasagna Stacks 75

6. Air-Fried Cajun Tilapia with Veggie Medley 76

7. Air-Fried Stuffed Bell Peppers 77

8. Air-Fried Garlic Herb Chicken Thighs 78

9. Air-Fried Ratatouille 79

10. Air-Fried Lemon Herb Cod 80

11. Air-Fried Greek Chicken with Veggies 81

    12. Air-Fried Cabbage Steaks 82

    13. Air-Fried Spaghetti Squash with Tomato Basil Sauce 83

    14. Air-Fried Asian-Inspired Salmon 83

    15. Air-Fried Portobello Mushroom Burgers........................... 84

CHAPTER FIVE 87

    Zero Point Air Fryer Snacks 87

    1. Air-Fried Zucchini Chips.. 87

    2. Air-Fried Spiced Chickpeas... 88

    3. Air-Fried Apple Slices with Cinnamon 89

    4. Air-Fried Buffalo Cauliflower Bites.................................... 89

    5. Air-Fried Eggplant Fries 90

    6. Air-Fried Kale Chips... 91

    7. Air-Fried Bell Pepper Nachos... 91

    8. Air-Fried Carrot Fries 92

    9. Air-Fried Edamame 93

    10. Air-Fried Radish Chips 94

CHAPTER SIX.. 95

    Zero Point Air Fryer Dessert... 95

    1. Air-Fried Cinnamon Apples 95

    2. Air-Fried Banana Slices with Cocoa Dusting...................... 95

3. Air-Fried Pineapple Rings 96

4. Air-Fried Pear Halves with Nutmeg 97

5. Air-Fried Peaches with Cinnamon and Vanilla 97

6. Air-Fried Grapefruit with Cinnamon Sugar Alternative....... 98

7. Air-Fried Mango Slices.. 99

9. Air-Fried Stuffed Apples with Date Filling 100

10. Air-Fried Strawberry "Shortcakes" 101

CONCLUSION 103

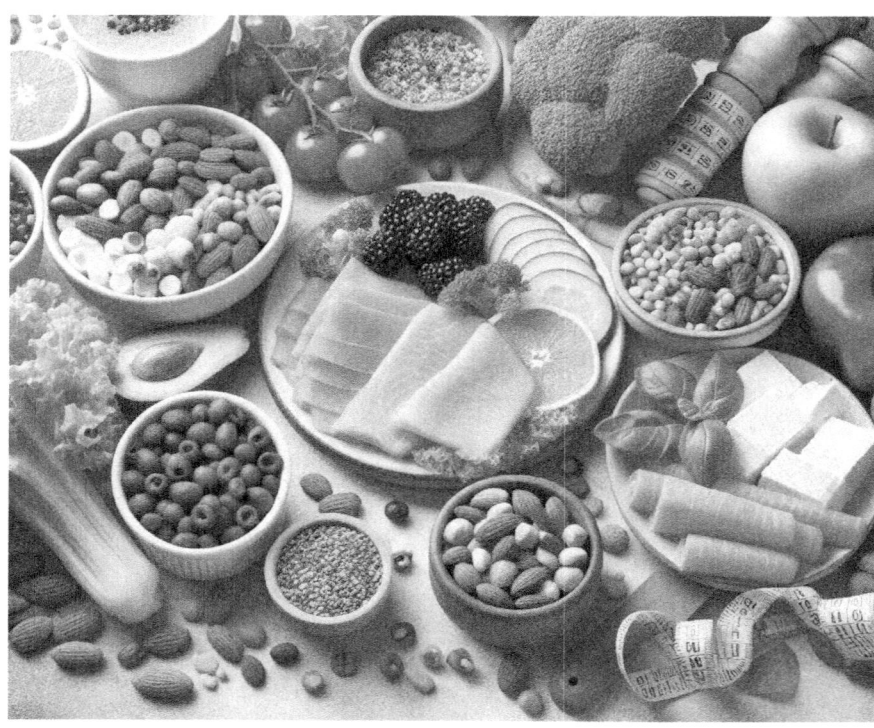

Introduction to The Zero Point Air Fryer Cookbook

Crispy, Delicious, and Guilt-Free Cooking Made Easy

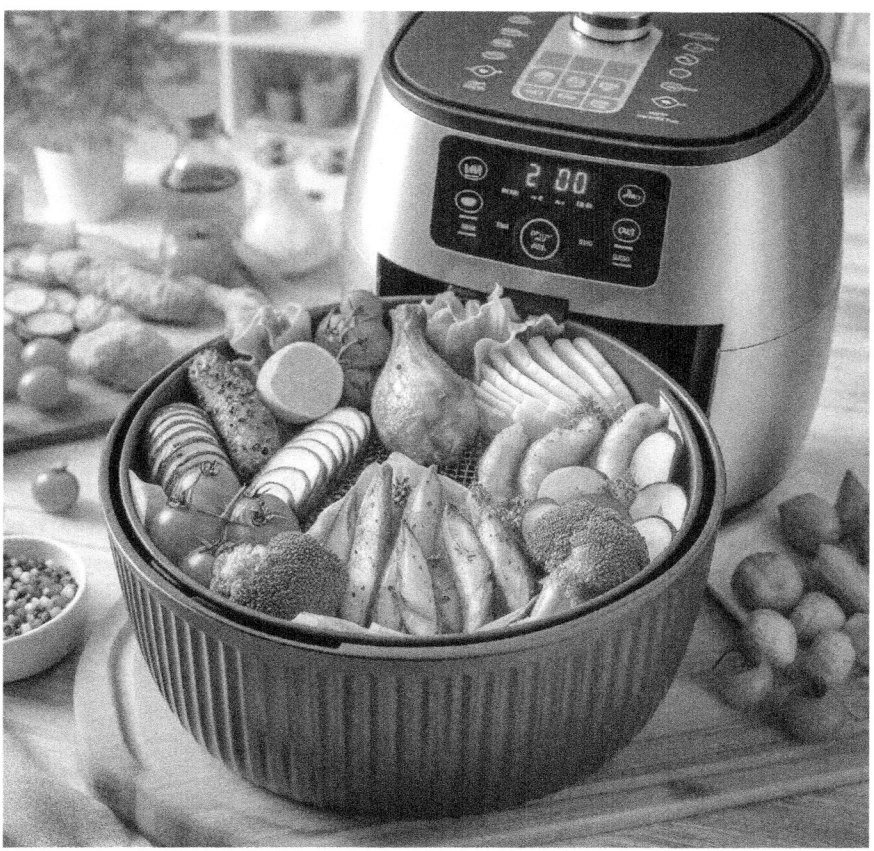

Imagine enjoying all your favorite crispy, crunchy dishes without the extra calories, guilt, or complicated cooking methods. Sounds like a dream, right? Well, your dream just came true!

Welcome to The Zero Point Air Fryer Cookbook 2025, your ultimate guide to mastering the art of healthy, flavorful, and zero-stress cooking with the magic of zero-point foods and your trusty air fryer.

Why This Cookbook?

If you've ever wished for a way to indulge in your favorite fried foods while sticking to your weight loss or wellness goals, this book is for you. The air fryer is a game-changer, allowing you to create healthier versions of your go-to comfort foods with little to no oil. Combined with the zero-point food philosophy, this cookbook empowers you to enjoy satisfying meals that keep you on track.

This isn't just a cookbook—it's your companion to a healthier lifestyle that doesn't compromise on taste or texture. Whether you're a seasoned air fryer user or a curious beginner, you'll find this book packed with insights, tips, and recipes that transform everyday ingredients into culinary masterpieces.

What You'll Learn

In The Zero Point Air Fryer Cookbook 2025, we go beyond just recipes. You'll learn:

- **The Basics of Zero-Point Foods:** Understand the concept of zero-point foods and how they fit into a balanced diet.

- **Mastering Your Air Fryer:** Get the most out of your air fryer with tips, tricks, and cooking hacks for perfect results every time.

- **Healthy Cooking Techniques:** Discover how to create crispy textures and bold flavors without relying on heavy oils, breading, or excess calories.

- **Meal Planning Made Simple:** Learn how to integrate zero-point air fryer recipes into your daily routine for effortless meal prep and planning.

What's Inside?

This cookbook is packed with mouthwatering recipes for every meal and occasion, including:

- **Breakfast:** Start your day with golden, fluffy air-fried eggs or a satisfying veggie hash.

- **Lunch:** Enjoy hearty options like air-fried salmon or crispy zucchini fritters.

- **Snacks:** Crave-worthy treats like spiced chickpeas and crunchy kale chips.

- **Dinner:** From roasted chicken to stuffed bell peppers, these recipes are guaranteed to impress.

- **Desserts:** Yes, even desserts! Indulge in air-fried apple chips or a guilt-free fruit crumble.

Who Is This Book For?

Whether you're focused on weight loss, exploring a healthier way of eating, or simply want to make the most of your air fryer, this book is for you. It's perfect for:

- **Beginners:** Easy-to-follow recipes and step-by-step instructions make this the ideal guide for anyone new to zero-point foods or air frying.

- **Busy Home Cooks:** Quick, time-saving recipes that fit into any schedule.

- **Health Enthusiasts:** Stay on track with flavorful, nutrient-rich meals.

- **Food Lovers:** Satisfy your cravings without compromising on taste or texture.

Get Ready to Transform Your Kitchen

With The Zero Point Air Fryer Cookbook 2025, healthy eating has never been this satisfying, simple, or exciting. Say goodbye to bland "diet food" and hello to vibrant, crunchy, and flavorful meals you'll love.

Are you ready to unlock the full potential of your air fryer and create meals that make you feel amazing inside and out? Let's get started—your journey to guilt-free indulgence begins here!

What Exactly is Zero Point Air Fryer Recipes

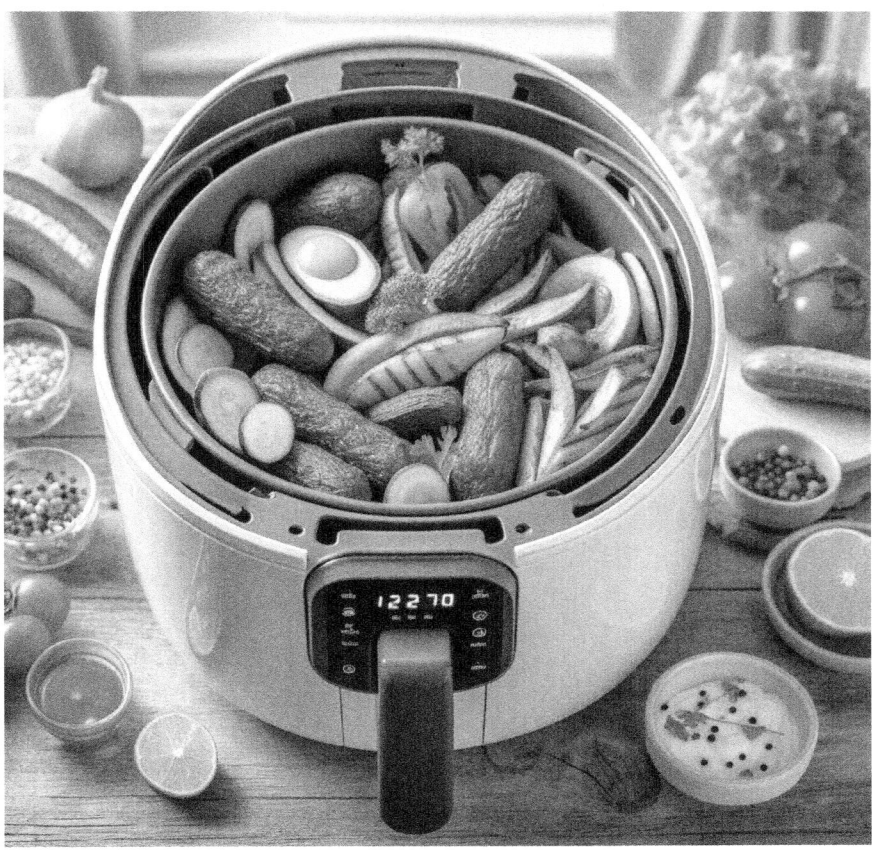

Zero Point Air Fryer Recipes refer to meals or snacks prepared using zero-point foods in an air fryer. These recipes are particularly useful for those following a weight loss plan, such as the WW (formerly Weight Watchers) program, where zero-point foods don't count toward your daily points.

The air fryer adds a bonus—it allows you to cook with little to no oil, making it a healthier option for crispy and flavorful dishes.

Zero-point air fryer recipes focus on ingredients like vegetables, lean proteins (like skinless chicken or fish), and fruits, which are cooked in the air fryer without adding high-calorie oils, breading, or sauces. These recipes are perfect for guilt-free indulgence while keeping meals light and nutritious.

Examples of Zero-Point Air Fryer Recipes

Air-Fried Cauliflower Buffalo Bites

Toss cauliflower florets in a mix of zero-point hot sauce and spices, then air fry for a crispy, spicy snack.

Air-Fried Salmon Fillets

Marinate salmon in lemon, garlic, and herbs, then air fry for a flaky, tender main dish.

Air-Fried Zucchini Chips

Slice zucchini into thin rounds, season with garlic powder and paprika, and air fry for a crunchy, low-calorie snack.

Air-Fried Apples with Cinnamon

Slice apples, sprinkle with cinnamon, and air fry for a warm, sweet treat.

Air-Fried Chicken Breast

Coat chicken breast with herbs and spices, air fry for a crispy, golden finish without breading or oil.

Benefits of Zero-Point Air Fryer Recipes

Low in Calories: Zero-point foods + air frying = guilt-free meals.

Time-Saving: Air fryers cook food quickly, making them ideal for busy days.

Crispy Texture: Achieve the crunch and flavor of fried foods without unhealthy fats.

Customizable: Easily adapt recipes to include your favorite zero-point ingredients.

How to Use an Air Fryer with Benefits

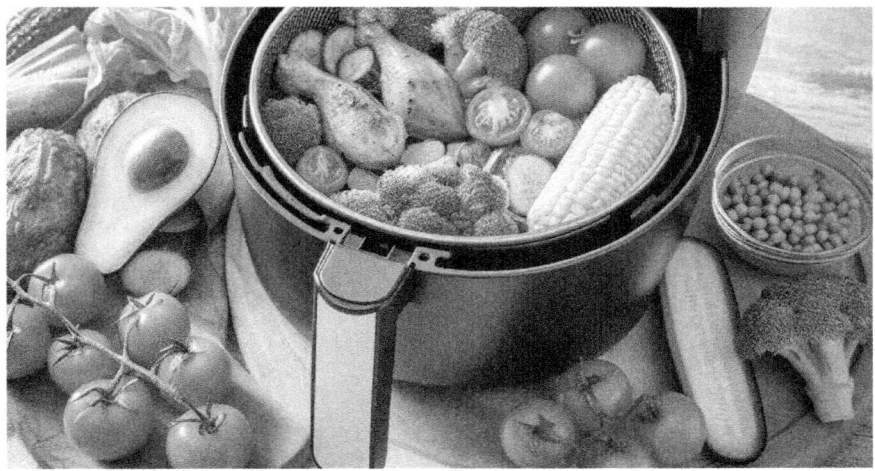

The air fryer is a kitchen revolution! With its ability to create crispy, delicious meals using little to no oil, it's no wonder it's become a favorite tool for healthy cooking. Whether you're a beginner or looking to make the most of your air fryer, here's a comprehensive guide to using it, along with the benefits it brings to your kitchen and lifestyle.

How to Use an Air Fryer

1. Get to Know Your Air Fryer:

- Parts to Identify: Most air fryers have a basket (where the food goes), a base unit with a heating element, and control settings.

- Settings: Familiarize yourself with temperature controls, timers, and pre-programmed cooking modes if available.

2. Preheat the Air Fryer (If Needed):

- Some air fryers recommend preheating for better results. Set it to the desired temperature and let it heat for 3–5 minutes.

3. Prepare Your Ingredients:

- Cut Evenly: Slice your food into uniform sizes for even cooking.

- Season Smartly: Toss your ingredients in spices or a light coating of oil if desired. For zero-point recipes, stick to seasoning blends or oil alternatives.

4. Load the Basket:

- Place food in a single layer for the crispiest results. Avoid overcrowding as this can prevent even airflow.

5. Set the Temperature and Time:

- Common cooking temperatures range from 325°F to 400°F (163°C to 204°C). Most recipes take 10–25 minutes, depending on the food.

6. Shake or Flip Midway:

- For even cooking, shake the basket or flip the food halfway through the cooking time.

7. Clean After Use:

- Let the air fryer cool down, then clean the basket and tray with warm, soapy water. Wipe the base unit with a damp cloth.

Benefits of Using an Air Fryer

1. Healthier Cooking:

- Air fryers use hot air to create the crispy texture of fried foods with up to 80% less oil, making meals lower in calories and fat.

2. Versatility:

- Cook everything from fries and chicken to roasted vegetables, baked goods, and even desserts.

3. Time-Saving:

- Air fryers cook faster than traditional ovens, making them perfect for busy lifestyles.

4. Energy-Efficient:

- Smaller than conventional ovens, they use less energy while delivering similar results.

5. Easy Cleanup:

- Nonstick baskets and detachable trays make cleaning quick and straightforward.

6. Flavorful Results:

- Achieve golden, crispy textures and rich flavors without the need for deep frying.

7. Safe and Convenient:

- Built-in timers, automatic shut-off, and cool-touch handles make air fryers user-friendly and safe for all.

Pro Tips for Air Fryer Success

- **Use the Right Oil:** If needed, a light spray of olive, avocado, or coconut oil works best. Avoid aerosol sprays, which can damage the basket.

- **Experiment with Accessories:** Consider investing in air fryer racks, pans, or skewers to expand your cooking options.

- **Don't Skip Maintenance:** Regular cleaning prevents food buildup and extends your air fryer's life.

Top Benefits of Air Fryer Cooking on Your Health

The air fryer has revolutionized how we approach cooking, offering a healthier alternative to traditional frying methods while preserving taste and texture. Here's how air fryer cooking can positively impact your health:

1. Reduced Fat and Calorie Intake

Traditional frying methods submerge food in oil, significantly increasing fat content and calories. Air fryers use hot air circulation to achieve a similar crispy texture with little to no oil.

- Health Impact: Lower fat consumption can reduce the risk of heart disease, obesity, and high cholesterol.

2. Lower Risk of Harmful Compounds

Deep frying can produce harmful compounds like acrylamide, which is linked to cancer risk. Air frying significantly reduces acrylamide formation while still delivering the crunch you love.

- Health Impact: Safer cooking methods contribute to long-term well-being and disease prevention.

3. Preserves Nutrients

Compared to frying or boiling, air frying retains more nutrients in vegetables and proteins because it requires shorter cooking times and minimal water usage.

- Health Impact: Nutrient-rich meals support immune health, energy levels, and overall vitality.

4. Supports Weight Loss Goals

Air fryer recipes often align with low-calorie or low-fat diets, helping you enjoy indulgent foods like fries or wings in a healthier way.

- Health Impact: Reducing calorie intake without sacrificing flavor aids in sustainable weight management.

5. Promotes Balanced Eating

The air fryer is versatile and encourages cooking from scratch, allowing you to include wholesome, minimally processed ingredients in your meals.

- Health Impact: Minimizing processed foods can lower sodium and additive intake, reducing the risk of hypertension and inflammation.

6. Encourages Portion Control

Cooking in an air fryer naturally limits batch sizes, helping with portion control and reducing overeating.

- Health Impact: Proper portions contribute to better digestion and balanced blood sugar levels.

7. Provides Allergy-Friendly Cooking

Air fryers are ideal for preparing allergen-free meals by avoiding cross-contamination in shared fryers or frying oil in restaurants.

- Health Impact: Safer cooking options for individuals with food allergies or sensitivities.

8. Supports a Low-Oil Diet

For people managing conditions like high cholesterol or gallbladder issues, reducing oil in cooking is essential. Air frying allows you to enjoy fried foods while adhering to dietary restrictions.

- Health Impact: A low-oil diet can improve heart health and reduce inflammation.

9. Convenient Healthy Eating

Air fryers are user-friendly, quick, and easy to clean, making it more appealing to prepare meals at home instead of relying on high-calorie takeout.

- Health Impact: Home-cooked meals are typically lower in salt, sugar, and unhealthy fats, promoting better overall health.

10. Encourages Creativity in Cooking

Using an air fryer inspires people to explore healthy ingredients like lean proteins, vegetables, and whole grains, leading to more balanced and diverse diets.

- Health Impact: Variety in your diet ensures you get essential nutrients for optimal health.

Final Thought

Switching to air fryer cooking isn't just a trend—it's a smart choice for your health. It allows you to enjoy your favorite foods in a way that supports your well-being while reducing health risks associated with traditional frying methods. With benefits ranging from weight management to reduced harmful compounds, air frying is a step toward a healthier, more delicious lifestyle!

With an air fryer, you can revolutionize your cooking routine, create healthier meals, and save time—all while enjoying delicious, crispy results. So, plug in your air fryer, gather your ingredients, and let the hot air work its magic!

CHAPTER ONE

Zero Point Meal Planning: A Guide to Healthy, Guilt-Free Eating

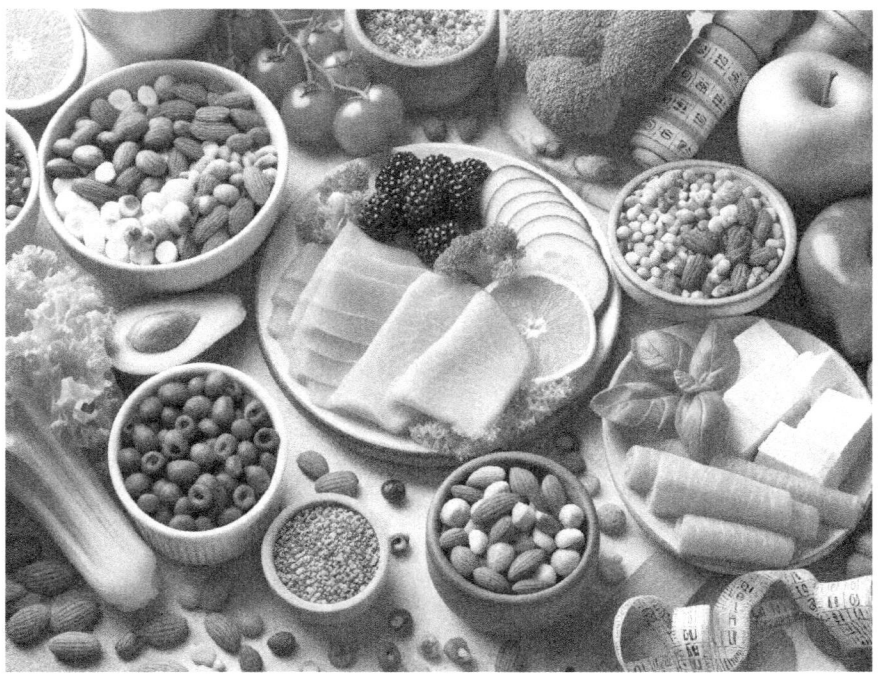

Meal planning with zero-point foods is an incredible way to stay on track with your health or weight loss goals while enjoying satisfying and flavorful meals. Whether you're following a weight-loss program or just looking to eat lighter and healthier, zero-point meal planning can help simplify your routine while keeping meals exciting and nutritious.

What Are Zero Point Foods?

Zero-point foods are those that don't need to be "counted" in certain diet plans because they are low in calories and nutrient-dense.

These foods are designed to be the building blocks of a healthy diet and often include:

- Vegetables: Broccoli, spinach, carrots, zucchini

- Fruits: Apples, berries, oranges

- Lean Proteins: Skinless chicken breast, turkey, eggs, tofu

- Legumes: Black beans, lentils, chickpeas

- Non-Fat Dairy: Plain Greek yogurt, cottage cheese

Benefits of Zero Point Meal Planning

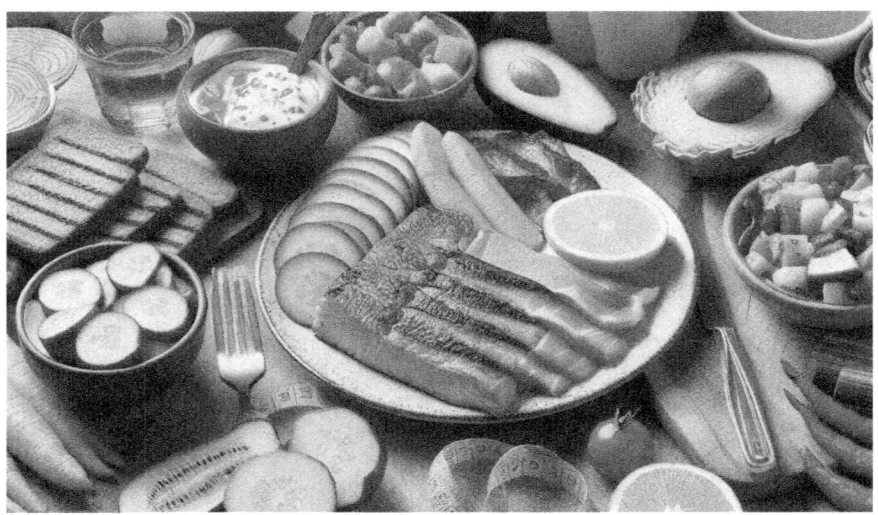

1. Simplifies Meal Tracking: No need to measure or weigh zero-point foods.

2. Encourages Healthy Choices: Focus on nutrient-rich, whole foods.

3. Boosts Satisfaction: Eat larger portions of zero-point foods without guilt.

4. Reduces Calorie Intake Naturally: Filling up on zero-point foods helps prevent overeating.

How to Start a Zero Point Meal Plan

Step 1: Start with a Framework

Plan your meals around three main components:

1. Protein: Build meals with lean, zero-point protein sources like eggs, chicken breast, or legumes.

2. Vegetables: Incorporate a variety of colorful, non-starchy veggies.

3. Flavor Boosters: Use spices, herbs, and zero-point sauces to keep meals exciting.

Step 2: Plan for All Meals

- **Breakfast:** Choose energizing options like veggie omelets, fruit smoothies, or non-fat yogurt with berries.

- **Lunch:** Opt for hearty salads, veggie-packed soups, or protein bowls.

- **Dinner:** Go for grilled fish, stir-fries, or roasted veggies with a lean protein source.

- **Snacks:** Keep cut fruits, veggies, or air-popped popcorn on hand for quick, guilt-free bites.

Step 3: Batch Cook and Prep

Batch cooking helps you stay on track during busy weeks. Prepare soups, roasted veggies, or grilled proteins in advance and portion them out for easy grab-and-go meals.

Step 4: Mix and Match

Create variety by mixing different zero-point foods throughout the week. For instance:

- Swap chicken breast for salmon.

- Change up your veggies by rotating broccoli, zucchini, or bell peppers.

- Add fruit toppings to yogurt or oatmeal for a sweet twist.

Pro Tips for Zero Point Meal Planning

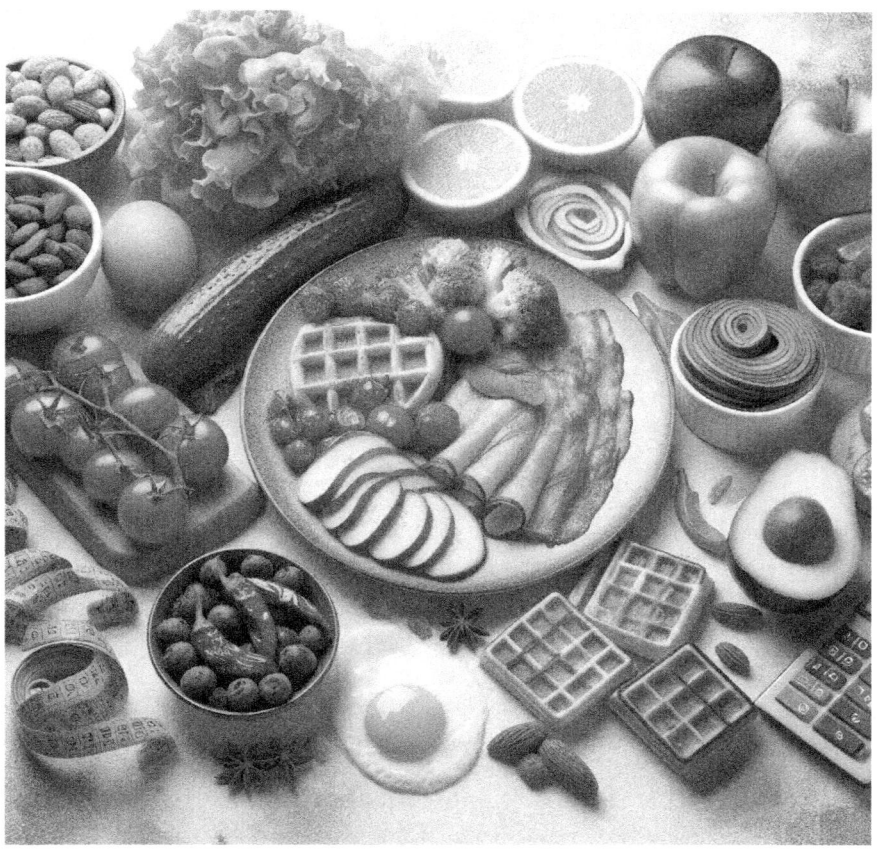

1. Prioritize Variety: Rotate your ingredients to avoid meal fatigue.

2. Watch for Hidden Calories: Be mindful of added oils, dressings, or sauces.

3. Stay Hydrated: Drink plenty of water to complement your healthy eating habits.

4. Keep It Balanced: While zero-point foods are amazing, ensure your diet includes healthy fats and whole grains in moderation for optimal nutrition.

Why Zero Point Meal Planning Works

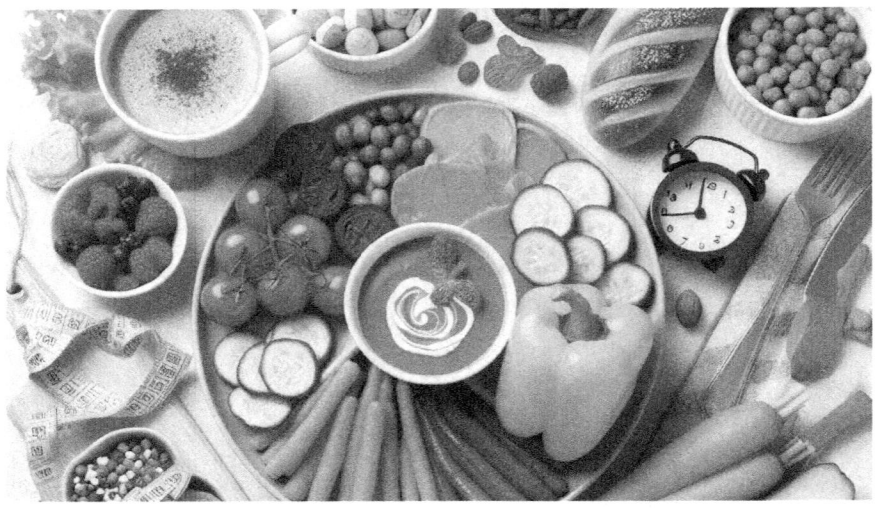

Zero-point meal planning empowers you to eat freely and enjoy your meals without the stress of calorie counting or guilt.

It's a practical, sustainable approach to building a healthy lifestyle, whether you're focused on weight loss, maintenance, or simply living well.

Start planning today, and discover how easy and enjoyable healthy eating can be!

CHAPTER ONE

14 Day Zero Point Air Fryer Meal Planning Recipes

Here's a complete 14-day Zero Point Air Fryer Meal Plan with unique recipes for each day, covering breakfast, lunch, and dinner. All recipes use zero-point ingredients, making it easy to stay on track with your health goals while enjoying tasty, crispy meals.

Week 1: Zero Point Air Fryer Meal Plan

Day 1

- Breakfast: Air-Fried Veggie Frittata Cups

  Ingredients: Eggs, spinach, bell peppers, onions.

  Instructions: Whisk eggs with diced veggies, pour into silicone cups, and air fry at 350°F for 12 minutes.

- Lunch: Air-Fried Lemon Herb Salmon

  Ingredients: Salmon fillet, lemon juice, parsley.

  Instructions: Marinate salmon, air fry at 375°F for 10 minutes.

- Dinner: Air-Fried Spiced Cauliflower and Chicken

  Ingredients: Cauliflower florets, paprika, cumin, chicken breast.

Instructions: Toss cauliflower in spices, air fry at 375°F for 15 minutes, and grill chicken.

Day 2

- Breakfast: Air-Fried Apple Slices with Cinnamon

Ingredients: Apple slices, cinnamon.

Instructions: Toss apples with cinnamon, air fry at 350°F for 10 minutes.

- Lunch: Crispy Chickpea Salad Wraps

Ingredients: Chickpeas, romaine lettuce, tomatoes.

Instructions: Air fry seasoned chickpeas at 400°F for 12 minutes, and wrap in lettuce with veggies.

- Dinner: Air-Fried Turkey Meatballs and Zucchini Noodles

Ingredients: Ground turkey, garlic, parsley, spiralized zucchini.

Instructions: Air fry meatballs at 375°F for 10 minutes, serve on zucchini noodles.

Day 3

- Breakfast: Air-Fried Sweet Potato Hash

Ingredients: Sweet potato cubes, onions, peppers.

Instructions: Toss with spices, air fry at 400°F for 15 minutes.

- Lunch: Air-Fried Shrimp and Cucumber Salad

Ingredients: Shrimp, cucumber, lemon.

Instructions: Air fry shrimp at 375°F for 8 minutes, toss with cucumber and lemon.

- Dinner: Air-Fried Eggplant Parmesan Stacks

Ingredients: Eggplant slices, tomato sauce, basil.

Instructions: Layer eggplant with sauce, air fry at 375°F for 12 minutes.

Day 4

- Breakfast: Air-Fried Berry Compote with Greek Yogurt

Ingredients: Blueberries, strawberries, Greek yogurt.

Instructions: Air fry berries at 350°F for 8 minutes, serve over yogurt.

- Lunch: Air-Fried Lemon Chicken Skewers

Ingredients: Chicken chunks, lemon juice, zucchini.

Instructions: Skewer and marinate chicken, air fry at 375°F for 12 minutes.

- Dinner: Air-Fried Tilapia with Asparagus

Ingredients: Tilapia, asparagus spears, garlic.

Instructions: Air fry tilapia and asparagus together at 375°F for 10 minutes.

Day 5

- Breakfast: Air-Fried Omelet Roll-Up

Ingredients: Eggs, spinach, diced peppers.

Instructions: Cook thin egg layers in the air fryer and roll with veggies.

- Lunch: Air-Fried Buffalo Cauliflower Bites

Ingredients: Cauliflower, buffalo sauce.

Instructions: Toss cauliflower with sauce, air fry at 375°F for 15 minutes.

- Dinner: Air-Fried Herb Turkey Patties with Mixed Veggies

Ingredients: Turkey patties, carrots, broccoli.

Instructions: Air fry patties at 375°F for 10 minutes, and veggies at 400°F for 8 minutes.

Day 6

- Breakfast: Air-Fried Grapefruit with Honey

  Ingredients: Grapefruit halves, honey, cinnamon.

  Instructions: Sprinkle grapefruit with honey and cinnamon, air fry at 375°F for 8 minutes.

- Lunch: Air-Fried Zucchini Chips and Turkey Wraps

  Ingredients: Zucchini, turkey slices, lettuce.

  Instructions: Air fry zucchini slices at 375°F for 10 minutes, serve with turkey wraps.

- Dinner: Air-Fried Garlic Shrimp and Green Beans

  Ingredients: Shrimp, green beans, garlic.

  Instructions: Air fry shrimp and beans together at 375°F for 10 minutes.

Day 7

- Breakfast: Air-Fried Banana Coins

  Ingredients: Banana slices, cinnamon.

  Instructions: Sprinkle banana slices with cinnamon, air fry at 350°F for 6 minutes.

- Lunch: Air-Fried Stuffed Bell Peppers

  Ingredients: Bell peppers, ground turkey, onions.

  Instructions: Stuff peppers, air fry at 375°F for 15 minutes.

- Dinner: Air-Fried Eggplant Lasagna

  Ingredients: Eggplant slices, tomato sauce, basil.

  Instructions: Layer eggplant with sauce, air fry at 375°F for 12 minutes.

Day 8

- Breakfast: Air-Fried Spinach and Mushroom Omelet

  Ingredients: Eggs, spinach, mushrooms.

  Instructions: Whisk eggs, pour into an air fryer-safe dish with sautéed spinach and mushrooms, air fry at 325°F for 8–10 minutes.

- Lunch: Air-Fried Lemon Garlic Shrimp with Roasted Asparagus

  Ingredients: Shrimp, asparagus, garlic, lemon.

  Instructions: Season shrimp and asparagus with garlic and lemon juice, air fry at 375°F for 10 minutes.

- Dinner: Air-Fried Turkey-Stuffed Zucchini Boats

  Ingredients: Zucchini, ground turkey, onions.

Instructions: Hollow out zucchini, stuff with cooked turkey mixture, air fry at 375°F for 15 minutes.

Day 9

- Breakfast: Air-Fried Tomato and Feta Egg Bake

  Ingredients: Eggs, cherry tomatoes, spinach, non-fat feta.

  Instructions: Combine ingredients in a ramekin, air fry at 325°F for 10 minutes.

- Lunch: Air-Fried Chicken and Veggie Skewers

  Ingredients: Chicken chunks, bell peppers, zucchini, onions.

  Instructions: Assemble skewers, season, and air fry at 375°F for 12 minutes.

- Dinner: Air-Fried Salmon Patties with Steamed Broccoli

  Ingredients: Salmon, egg, parsley, lemon.

  Instructions: Form patties, air fry at 375°F for 8 minutes, and serve with broccoli.

Day 10

- Breakfast: Air-Fried Apple Chips with Cinnamon

  Ingredients: Apple slices, cinnamon.

Instructions: Thinly slice apples, sprinkle with cinnamon, and air fry at 350°F for 10 minutes.

- Lunch: Air-Fried Turkey and Spinach Wraps

Ingredients: Ground turkey, spinach leaves, romaine lettuce.

Instructions: Cook turkey in the air fryer at 375°F for 8 minutes, wrap with spinach and lettuce.

- Dinner: Air-Fried Eggplant Parmesan

Ingredients: Eggplant, tomato sauce, basil.

Instructions: Layer eggplant slices with sauce, air fry at 375°F for 12 minutes.

Day 11

- Breakfast: Air-Fried Berry French Toast (Zero Point Style)

Ingredients: Egg, whole-grain bread (optional), mixed berries.

Instructions: Dip bread in whisked egg, air fry at 350°F for 8 minutes, and top with berries.

- Lunch: Air-Fried Tofu Stir-Fry with Snap Peas

Ingredients: Firm tofu, snap peas, soy sauce.

Instructions: Cube tofu, air fry at 375°F for 10 minutes, and toss with stir-fried snap peas.

- Dinner: Air-Fried Lemon Garlic Cod with Roasted Carrots

  Ingredients: Cod fillets, garlic, lemon, carrots.

  Instructions: Season cod and carrots, air fry at 375°F for 12 minutes.

Day 12

- Breakfast: Air-Fried Banana and Oat Pancakes

  Ingredients: Mashed bananas, oats, eggs.

  Instructions: Mix ingredients, form pancakes, and air fry on parchment paper at 350°F for 10 minutes.

- Lunch: Air-Fried Zucchini Chips with Salsa Dip

  Ingredients: Zucchini slices, paprika, salsa.

  Instructions: Toss zucchini with paprika, air fry at 375°F for 10 minutes, serve with salsa.

- Dinner: Air-Fried Turkey Burgers with Roasted Bell Peppers

  Ingredients: Ground turkey, garlic, bell peppers.

  Instructions: Form turkey patties, air fry at 375°F for 8 minutes, and roast peppers alongside.

Day 13

- Breakfast: Air-Fried Hard-Boiled Eggs and Cucumber Slices

Ingredients: Whole eggs, cucumbers.

Instructions: Air fry eggs at 250°F for 15 minutes, and serve with cucumber slices.

- Lunch: Air-Fried Shrimp Tacos with Lettuce Wraps

Ingredients: Shrimp, lettuce leaves, diced tomatoes.

Instructions: Air fry shrimp at 375°F for 8 minutes, and serve in lettuce wraps with tomatoes.

- Dinner: Air-Fried Chicken Drumsticks with Broccoli

Ingredients: Chicken drumsticks (skinless), garlic, broccoli florets.

Instructions: Season chicken and broccoli, air fry at 375°F for 15 minutes.

Day 14

- Breakfast: Air-Fried Sweet Potato Toast with Avocado

Ingredients: Sweet potato slices, mashed avocado.

Instructions: Slice sweet potato into "toast," air fry at 375°F for 10 minutes, and top with avocado.

- Lunch: Air-Fried Chickpea and Spinach Salad

Ingredients: Chickpeas, spinach, lemon juice.

Instructions: Air fry chickpeas at 400°F for 10 minutes, and toss with spinach and lemon juice.

- Dinner: Air-Fried Tilapia with Roasted Green Beans

Ingredients: Tilapia fillet, green beans, lemon.

Instructions: Season tilapia and beans, air fry at 375°F for 10 minutes.

Tips for Success:

1. Prep Ahead: Chop and marinate ingredients the night before to save time.

2. Rotate Ingredients: Swap proteins and veggies to keep meals diverse.

3. Balance Flavors: Use herbs, spices, and citrus to enhance taste without extra calories.

This complete 14-day Zero Point Air Fryer Meal Plan offers a satisfying and healthy variety of meals, proving that eating light doesn't have to mean sacrificing flavor or convenience!

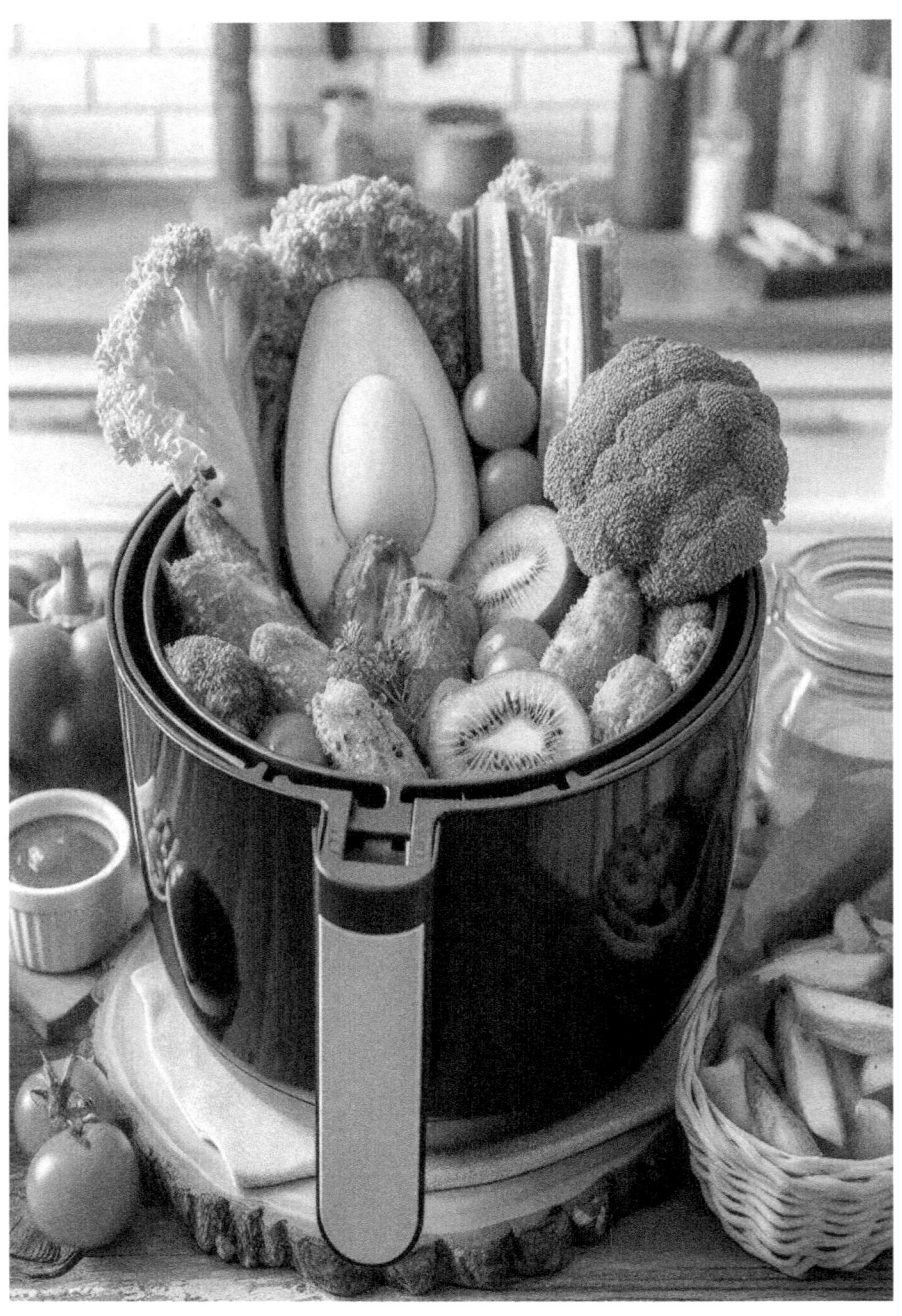

CHAPTER TWO

Zero Point Air Fryer Breakfast Recipes

1. Air-Fried Veggie Egg Cups

Ingredients:

- 2 large eggs (zero points on certain programs)

- 1/4 cup bell peppers, diced

- 1/4 cup spinach, chopped

- Salt and pepper to taste

Instructions:

1. Preheat the air fryer to 350°F.

2. In a bowl, whisk the eggs and season with salt and pepper.

3. Add the diced bell peppers and spinach to the egg mixture.

4. Pour the mixture into silicone muffin cups or an air fryer-safe pan.

5. Air fry for 8-10 minutes, or until the eggs are set.

6. Let cool for a minute before serving. These are perfect for meal prep too!

2. Air-Fried Sweet Potato Hash

Ingredients:

- 1 medium sweet potato, peeled and diced

- 1/4 cup onion, diced

- 1/4 cup bell pepper, diced

- 1 tsp paprika

- Salt and pepper to taste

Instructions:

1. Preheat the air fryer to 375°F.

2. Toss the diced sweet potatoes, onion, and bell pepper with paprika, salt, and pepper.

3. Spread the mixture evenly in the air fryer basket.

4. Air fry for 15-20 minutes, shaking the basket halfway through.

5. Serve as is or top with your favorite zero-point sauce for extra flavor.

3. Air-Fried Banana Pancakes (Zero Point Style)

Ingredients:

- 1 ripe banana, mashed

- 1 egg

- 1/2 tsp vanilla extract

- Cinnamon to taste

- 1/4 tsp baking powder

Instructions:

1. Preheat the air fryer to 350°F.

2. In a bowl, mash the banana and mix with the egg, vanilla, cinnamon, and baking powder.

3. Spoon small dollops of the mixture onto parchment paper, forming pancake shapes.

4. Place the parchment paper into the air fryer basket.

5. Air fry for 8 minutes or until golden brown.

6. Serve with fresh fruit or a drizzle of sugar-free syrup.

4. Air-Fried Apple Cinnamon Chips

Ingredients:

- 2 medium apples, thinly sliced

- 1/2 tsp cinnamon

- A pinch of salt

Instructions:

1. Preheat the air fryer to 350°F.

2. Slice the apples thinly and sprinkle with cinnamon and salt.

3. Arrange the apple slices in a single layer in the air fryer basket.

4. Air fry for 10 minutes, flipping halfway through.

5. Once crispy, remove and let cool for a few minutes. These chips are sweet, crunchy, and perfect for breakfast or a snack!

5. Air-Fried Breakfast Quesadilla

Ingredients:

- 2 small whole-wheat tortillas

- 1/4 cup egg whites

- 1/4 cup bell pepper, diced

- 1/4 cup spinach, chopped

- Salsa (optional)

Instructions:

1. Preheat the air fryer to 350°F.

2. Scramble the egg whites with diced bell pepper and spinach.

3. Place the mixture between two tortillas.

4. Air fry for 5-6 minutes, flipping halfway through.

5. Once crispy and golden, remove and slice into wedges. Serve with salsa on the side for an extra kick!

6. Air-Fried Avocado Toast (Zero Point Style)

Ingredients:

- 1 slice whole grain bread (check for zero-point options based on your program)

- 1/2 avocado, mashed

- Salt and pepper to taste

- Red pepper flakes (optional)

Instructions:

1. Preheat the air fryer to 350°F.

2. Place the bread in the air fryer and toast for 4–5 minutes until golden and crisp.

3. While the bread is toasting, mash the avocado in a bowl and season with salt, pepper, and red pepper flakes.

4. Once the toast is ready, spread the mashed avocado on top.

5. Enjoy as a simple, satisfying breakfast!

7. Air-Fried Apple Cinnamon Oats

Ingredients:

- 1/2 cup rolled oats

- 1 medium apple, peeled and diced

- 1/2 tsp cinnamon

- 1/4 tsp vanilla extract

- 1/4 cup water

Instructions:

1. Preheat the air fryer to 350°F.

2. In a small bowl, mix the oats, diced apple, cinnamon, vanilla extract, and water.

3. Pour the mixture into a small oven-safe dish or ramekin.

4. Place the dish in the air fryer and cook for 12–15 minutes, stirring halfway through.

5. Once the oats are soft and the apples are tender, remove and serve warm.

8. Air-Fried Veggie Frittata Bites

Ingredients:

- 2 large egg whites

- 1/4 cup zucchini, diced

- 1/4 cup bell peppers, diced

- 1/4 cup onions, diced

- Salt and pepper to taste

Instructions:

1. Preheat the air fryer to 350°F.

2. Whisk the egg whites and season with salt and pepper.

3. Stir in the diced zucchini, bell peppers, and onions.

4. Pour the mixture into silicone muffin cups or an air fryer-safe pan.

5. Air fry for 10–12 minutes, or until the egg bites are fully cooked.

6. Let cool for a minute and enjoy these delicious veggie-packed frittata bites!

9. Air-Fried Breakfast Stuffed Peppers

Ingredients:

- 2 bell peppers, halved and seeded

- 2 egg whites

- 1/4 cup spinach, chopped

- Salt and pepper to taste

- 1/4 tsp garlic powder (optional)

Instructions:

1. Preheat the air fryer to 375°F.

2. Crack the egg whites into a bowl, add the spinach, salt, pepper, and garlic powder, and mix well.

3. Stuff each bell pepper half with the egg mixture.

4. Place the stuffed peppers in the air fryer basket and air fry for 10–12 minutes, until the eggs are set.

5. Let cool slightly, then enjoy these healthy, stuffed bell pepper breakfasts!

10. Air-Fried Zucchini Boats with Eggs

Ingredients:

- 2 medium zucchinis, halved and scooped out

- 2 egg whites

- 1/4 cup tomatoes, diced

- Salt, pepper, and Italian seasoning to taste

Instructions:

1. Preheat the air fryer to 375°F.

2. Scoop out the zucchini halves and season with salt, pepper, and Italian seasoning.

3. Fill each zucchini boat with egg whites and top with diced tomatoes.

4. Air fry for 10–12 minutes, until the eggs are cooked through and the zucchini is tender.

5. Serve as a light yet filling breakfast packed with protein and veggies!

11. Air-Fried Breakfast Veggie Quesadilla

Ingredients:

- 2 small corn tortillas (check for zero points)

- 1/2 cup bell peppers, diced

- 1/4 cup onions, diced

- 1/2 cup spinach, chopped

- Salt and pepper to taste

Instructions:

1. Preheat the air fryer to 350°F.

2. Sauté the bell peppers, onions, and spinach in a pan until tender (optional).

3. Layer one tortilla with the sautéed veggies and place the second tortilla on top.

4. Air fry for 5–6 minutes, flipping halfway through.

5. Slice and serve with salsa or Greek yogurt for a tasty and filling breakfast!

12. Air-Fried French Toast Sticks (Zero Point Style)

Ingredients:

- 2 slices whole-grain bread (or any zero-point bread option)

- 1 egg white

- 1 tsp cinnamon

- 1/4 tsp vanilla extract

- 1/4 cup unsweetened almond milk

Instructions:

1. Preheat the air fryer to 375°F.

2. In a shallow bowl, whisk the egg white, almond milk, cinnamon, and vanilla extract.

3. Cut the bread into strips and dip each strip into the egg mixture.

4. Place the bread strips in the air fryer basket in a single layer and air fry for 8–10 minutes, flipping halfway through.

5. Serve with fresh fruit or sugar-free syrup for a delicious and zero-point breakfast.

13. Air-Fried Sweet Potato Breakfast Bites

Ingredients:

- 1 medium sweet potato, peeled and cubed

- 1/2 tsp cinnamon

- 1/4 tsp nutmeg

- 1 tbsp maple syrup (optional, or use sugar-free syrup for zero points)

Instructions:

1. Preheat the air fryer to 375°F.

2. Toss the sweet potato cubes with cinnamon, nutmeg, and a drizzle of maple syrup.

3. Air fry for 12–15 minutes, shaking the basket halfway through.

4. Once crispy and tender, serve these bites warm for a filling and naturally sweet breakfast.

14. Air-Fried Mini Breakfast Frittatas

Ingredients:

- 2 large egg whites

- 1/4 cup bell peppers, diced

- 1/4 cup mushrooms, diced

- 1/4 cup spinach, chopped

- Salt and pepper to taste

Instructions:

1. Preheat the air fryer to 350°F.

2. In a bowl, whisk the egg whites and season with salt and pepper.

3. Add in the diced bell peppers, mushrooms, and spinach.

4. Pour the mixture into silicone muffin cups or small ramekins.

5. Air fry for 8–10 minutes until the eggs are fully cooked.

6. Enjoy these mini frittatas as a protein-packed, veggie-filled breakfast!

15. Air-Fried Oatmeal Cups with Berries

Ingredients:

- 1/2 cup rolled oats

- 1/4 cup almond milk

- 1/2 tsp cinnamon

- 1/4 cup mixed berries (fresh or frozen)

- 1 tsp chia seeds (optional)

Instructions:

1. Preheat the air fryer to 350°F.

2. In a bowl, mix the rolled oats, almond milk, and cinnamon.

3. Spoon the mixture into silicone muffin cups, filling each cup about halfway.

4. Top with mixed berries and chia seeds (if using).

5. Air fry for 10–12 minutes, or until the oatmeal cups are golden and set.

6. Allow them to cool for a minute before enjoying these portable, zero-point oatmeal cups!

These Zero Point Air Fryer Breakfast Recipes continue to make your mornings delicious and nutritious, while keeping you on track with your healthy eating goals.

Whether you're craving sweet or savory, these recipes are versatile, quick, and full of flavor.

Enjoy!

CHAPTER THREE

Zero Point Air Fryer Lunch Recipes

1. Air-Fried Veggie Fajitas

Ingredients:

- 1/2 bell pepper, sliced

- 1/2 onion, sliced

- 1/4 zucchini, sliced

- 1/4 tsp chili powder

- 1/4 tsp cumin

- 1/4 tsp garlic powder

- Salt and pepper to taste

- 2 small corn tortillas (check for zero points)

Instructions:

1. Preheat the air fryer to 375°F.

2. Toss the bell pepper, onion, and zucchini with chili powder, cumin, garlic powder, salt, and pepper.

3. Air fry the vegetables for 10-12 minutes, shaking halfway through.

4. Warm the tortillas in the air fryer for 1-2 minutes.

5. Fill the tortillas with the air-fried veggies and serve with a squeeze of lime or salsa for added flavor.

2. Air-Fried Chickpea Salad Wrap

Ingredients:

- 1/2 cup canned chickpeas, drained and rinsed

- 1 tsp olive oil (optional for flavor)

- 1/4 tsp paprika

- 1/4 tsp garlic powder

- Salt and pepper to taste

- 1 large lettuce leaf or whole wheat wrap

- 1/4 cup diced cucumber

- 1/4 cup diced tomato

- 1/4 cup shredded carrots

Instructions:

1. Preheat the air fryer to 375°F.

2. Toss the chickpeas with olive oil (optional), paprika, garlic powder, salt, and pepper.

3. Air fry the chickpeas for 10-12 minutes, shaking halfway through, until crispy.

4. In a bowl, combine the diced cucumber, tomato, and shredded carrots.

5. Place the crispy chickpeas on the lettuce leaf or whole wheat wrap and top with the fresh veggies. Roll up and enjoy!

3. Air-Fried Cauliflower Steaks

Ingredients:

- 1 medium cauliflower, sliced into steaks

- 1 tsp olive oil (optional)

- 1/4 tsp garlic powder

- 1/4 tsp paprika

- Salt and pepper to taste

- Fresh parsley for garnish

Instructions:

1. Preheat the air fryer to 375°F.

2. Brush the cauliflower steaks with olive oil (optional) and season with garlic powder, paprika, salt, and pepper.

3. Air fry the cauliflower steaks for 10-12 minutes, flipping halfway through.

4. Once tender and golden, garnish with fresh parsley.

5. Serve as a main dish or as a side with your favorite zero-point sauce.

4. Air-Fried Veggie Burgers

Ingredients:

- 1/2 cup black beans, mashed

- 1/4 cup grated zucchini

- 1/4 cup chopped onions

- 1/4 cup breadcrumbs (use whole wheat for zero-point options)

- 1/4 tsp garlic powder

- Salt and pepper to taste

Instructions:

1. Preheat the air fryer to 375°F.

2. In a bowl, mix the mashed black beans, grated zucchini, chopped onions, breadcrumbs, garlic powder, salt, and pepper.

3. Form the mixture into patties.

4. Place the patties in the air fryer basket and cook for 8-10 minutes, flipping halfway through.

5. Serve the veggie burgers on a lettuce wrap or whole-grain bun, and top with your favorite toppings like tomatoes or pickles.

5. Air-Fried Stuffed Bell Peppers

Ingredients:

- 2 bell peppers, halved and seeded

- 1/2 cup cooked quinoa or brown rice (optional)

- 1/4 cup black beans

- 1/4 cup diced tomatoes

- 1/4 tsp cumin

- 1/4 tsp chili powder

- Salt and pepper to taste

Instructions:

1. Preheat the air fryer to 375°F.

2. In a bowl, mix the cooked quinoa or rice, black beans, diced tomatoes, cumin, chili powder, salt, and pepper.

3. Stuff the bell pepper halves with the mixture.

4. Air fry the stuffed peppers for 10-12 minutes until the peppers are tender and the filling is heated through.

5. Serve hot and enjoy as a filling, low-calorie lunch option!

6. Air-Fried Veggie Tacos

Ingredients:

- 1/2 cup zucchini, diced

- 1/2 cup bell pepper, diced

- 1/4 cup red onion, diced

- 1/4 tsp cumin

- 1/4 tsp chili powder

- Salt and pepper to taste

- 2 small corn tortillas (check for zero points)

- Salsa and lime for topping

Instructions:

1. Preheat the air fryer to 375°F.

2. Toss the zucchini, bell pepper, and onion with cumin, chili powder, salt, and pepper.

3. Air fry the veggies for 8-10 minutes, shaking the basket halfway through.

4. Warm the tortillas in the air fryer for 1-2 minutes.

5. Assemble the tacos by adding the air-fried veggies to the tortillas and topping with salsa and a squeeze of lime. Enjoy!

7. Air-Fried Falafel

Ingredients:

- 1/2 cup canned chickpeas, drained and rinsed

- 1/4 cup parsley, chopped

- 2 tbsp onion, finely chopped

- 1 garlic clove, minced

- 1/2 tsp cumin

- 1/4 tsp coriander

- Salt and pepper to taste

- 1 tbsp flour (optional, or use zero-point flour)

Instructions:

1. Preheat the air fryer to 375°F.

2. In a food processor, combine chickpeas, parsley, onion, garlic, cumin, coriander, salt, pepper, and flour (if using). Pulse until well combined but still chunky.

3. Shape the mixture into small balls or patties.

4. Air fry for 10-12 minutes, flipping halfway through, until golden and crispy.

5. Serve with a light tahini sauce or in a wrap for a tasty, satisfying lunch!

8. Air-Fried Sweet Potato Fries

Ingredients:

- 1 medium sweet potato, peeled and cut into fries

- 1 tsp olive oil (optional)

- 1/4 tsp paprika

- 1/4 tsp garlic powder

- Salt and pepper to taste

Instructions:

1. Preheat the air fryer to 375°F.

2. Toss the sweet potato fries with olive oil (optional), paprika, garlic powder, salt, and pepper.

3. Air fry for 12-15 minutes, shaking halfway through, until crispy and golden.

4. Serve with a side of your favorite dipping sauce or enjoy on their own as a healthy and filling lunch.

9. Air-Fried Portobello Mushroom Burgers

Ingredients:

- 2 large Portobello mushroom caps

- 1 tbsp balsamic vinegar

- 1/2 tsp garlic powder

- 1/4 tsp thyme

- Salt and pepper to taste

- Lettuce, tomato, and pickles for garnish

Instructions:

1. Preheat the air fryer to 375°F.

2. Brush the mushroom caps with balsamic vinegar, garlic powder, thyme, salt, and pepper.

3. Air fry the mushrooms for 8-10 minutes until tender.

4. Serve the mushrooms as "burger patties" on lettuce wraps, topped with tomato and pickles for a low-calorie, savory lunch.

10. Air-Fried Eggplant Parmesan

Ingredients:

- 1 small eggplant, sliced into rounds

- 1/4 cup breadcrumbs (use whole wheat or zero-point options)

- 1/4 cup marinara sauce (sugar-free)

- 1 tbsp Parmesan cheese (optional)

- Salt and pepper to taste

Instructions:

1. Preheat the air fryer to 375°F.

2. Dip the eggplant slices into the breadcrumbs, coating them evenly.

3. Air fry the eggplant for 8-10 minutes until crispy and golden.

4. Top each slice with a spoonful of marinara sauce and sprinkle with Parmesan cheese (optional).

5. Air fry for an additional 2-3 minutes until heated through.

6. Serve as a light, crispy, and satisfying lunch!

11. Air-Fried Stuffed Zucchini Boats

Ingredients:

- 2 medium zucchinis, halved and seeded

- 1/4 cup diced tomatoes

- 1/4 cup bell pepper, diced

- 1/4 cup onion, diced

- 1/4 tsp garlic powder

- 1/4 tsp Italian seasoning

- Salt and pepper to taste

- Fresh basil for garnish

Instructions:

1. Preheat the air fryer to 375°F.

2. Scoop out the center of each zucchini half to create boats.

3. In a bowl, combine diced tomatoes, bell pepper, onion, garlic powder, Italian seasoning, salt, and pepper.

4. Stuff the zucchini halves with the veggie mixture.

5. Air fry for 10-12 minutes until the zucchini is tender and the filling is heated through.

6. Garnish with fresh basil before serving for a fresh, flavorful lunch.

12. Air-Fried Veggie-Stuffed Mushrooms

Ingredients:

- 6 large mushrooms, stems removed

- 1/4 cup spinach, chopped

- 1/4 cup bell pepper, finely chopped

- 1 tbsp onions, finely chopped

- 1/4 tsp garlic powder

- Salt and pepper to taste

Instructions:

1. Preheat the air fryer to 375°F.

2. In a small bowl, combine spinach, bell pepper, onion, garlic powder, salt, and pepper.

3. Stuff the mushroom caps with the veggie mixture.

4. Place the stuffed mushrooms in the air fryer basket and cook for 8-10 minutes, or until tender.

5. Serve as a light and savory lunch option that's full of flavor and nutrients.

13. Air-Fried Spicy Tofu Bites

Ingredients:

- 1 block firm tofu, pressed and cut into cubes

- 1 tsp olive oil (optional)

- 1/2 tsp chili powder

- 1/4 tsp garlic powder

- 1/4 tsp smoked paprika

- Salt and pepper to taste

Instructions:

1. Preheat the air fryer to 375°F.

2. Toss the tofu cubes in olive oil (if using) and sprinkle with chili powder, garlic powder, smoked paprika, salt, and pepper.

3. Air fry for 10-12 minutes, shaking halfway through, until crispy.

4. Serve as a high-protein, plant-based lunch with a side of veggies or salad.

14. Air-Fried Avocado Toast

Ingredients:

- 1 slice whole-grain bread (check for zero points)

- 1/2 ripe avocado, mashed

- 1 tsp lemon juice

- Salt and pepper to taste

- Red pepper flakes for garnish (optional)

Instructions:

1. Preheat the air fryer to 375°F.

2. Toast the slice of bread in the air fryer for 3-5 minutes until crispy.

3. While the bread is toasting, mash the avocado with lemon juice, salt, and pepper.

4. Once the toast is ready, spread the mashed avocado on top.

5. Garnish with red pepper flakes for a spicy kick, and enjoy a quick, tasty, and filling lunch!

15. Air-Fried Veggie & Bean Wrap

Ingredients:

- 1 whole wheat wrap (zero-point option)

- 1/2 cup black beans, rinsed and drained

- 1/4 cup corn kernels

- 1/4 cup bell peppers, diced

- 1/4 cup lettuce, shredded

- 1/4 tsp cumin

- 1/4 tsp chili powder

- Salsa for dipping (optional)

Instructions:

1. Preheat the air fryer to 375°F.

2. In a bowl, combine black beans, corn, bell peppers, cumin, and chili powder.

3. Warm the whole wheat wrap in the air fryer for 1-2 minutes.

4. Place the veggie and bean mixture in the center of the wrap and top with shredded lettuce.

5. Roll up the wrap and return it to the air fryer for 3-4 minutes to crisp up the outside.

6. Serve with salsa for dipping, and enjoy a filling, nutritious, and low-calorie lunch!

These Zero Point Air Fryer Lunch Recipes are perfect for anyone looking to enjoy a healthy, satisfying, and zero-point lunch. From stuffed veggies to crispy tofu bites, these dishes are easy to prepare and full of flavor. Try them out and keep your meals exciting and on-track!

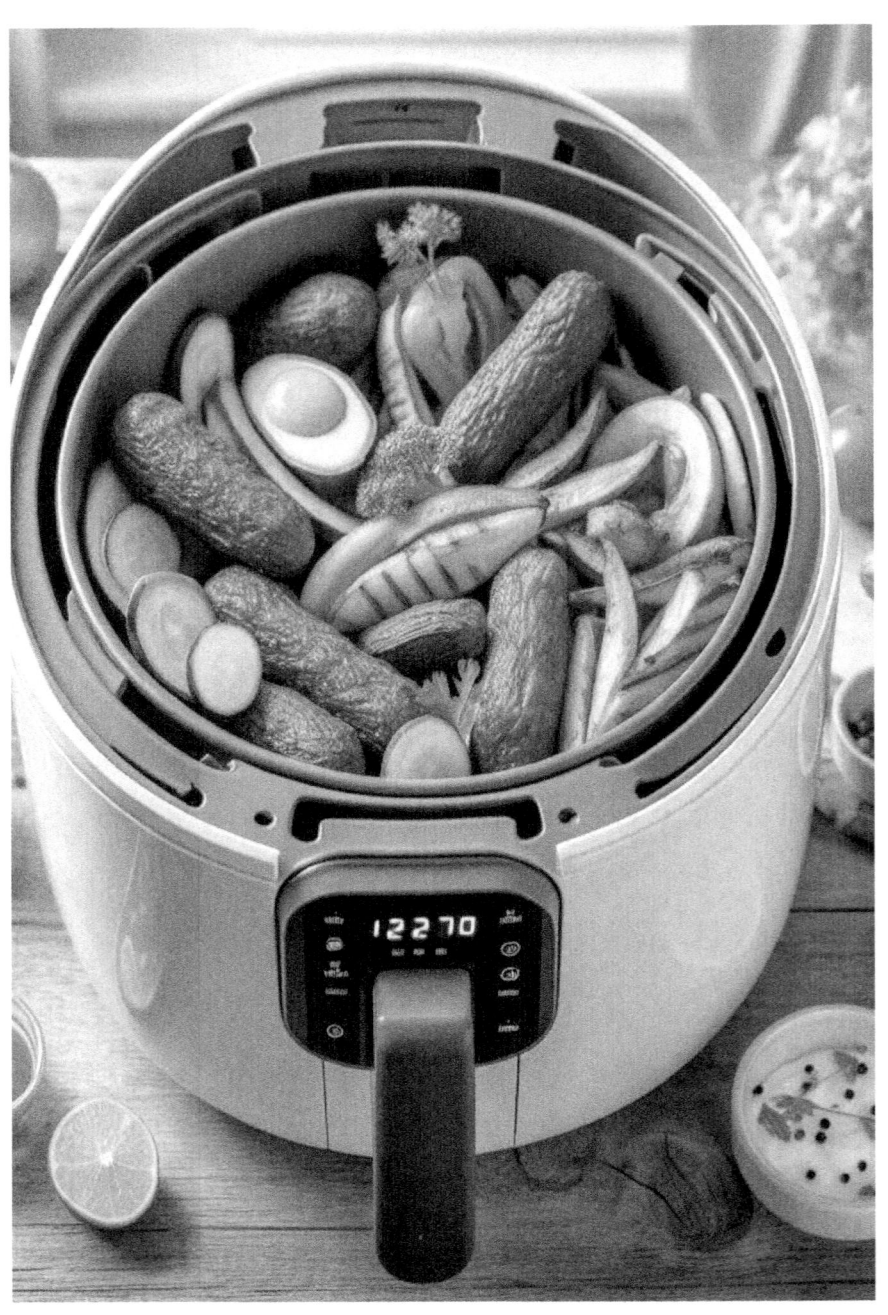

CHAPTER FOUR

Zero Point Air Fryer Dinner Recipes

1. Air-Fried Lemon Garlic Shrimp with Zoodles

Ingredients:

- 1 lb shrimp, peeled and deveined

- 2 zucchini, spiralized

- 1 lemon, juiced

- 2 garlic cloves, minced

- 1/4 tsp paprika

- Salt and pepper to taste

- Fresh parsley for garnish

Instructions:

1. Preheat the air fryer to 375°F.

2. In a bowl, toss the shrimp with lemon juice, garlic, paprika, salt, and pepper.

3. Air fry the shrimp for 6-8 minutes, shaking halfway through, until pink and cooked through.

4. While the shrimp cooks, sauté the zucchini noodles in a pan with a little lemon juice and garlic.

5. Serve the shrimp over the zoodles and garnish with fresh parsley.

2. Air-Fried Turkey Meatballs with Marinara Sauce

Ingredients:

- 1 lb lean ground turkey

- 1 egg white

- 1/4 cup onion, finely chopped

- 1/4 cup breadcrumbs (use zero-point options)

- 1/2 tsp Italian seasoning

- 1/4 tsp garlic powder

- Salt and pepper to taste

- 1/2 cup marinara sauce (sugar-free)

Instructions:

1. Preheat the air fryer to 375°F.

2. In a bowl, combine ground turkey, egg white, onion, breadcrumbs, Italian seasoning, garlic powder, salt, and pepper. Mix well and shape into small meatballs.

3. Air fry the meatballs for 10-12 minutes, shaking halfway through, until golden brown and cooked through.

4. Heat the marinara sauce and serve it over the meatballs for a hearty dinner.

3. Air-Fried Herb-Crusted Salmon

Ingredients:

- 2 salmon fillets (skin on or off)

- 1 tsp olive oil (optional)

- 1/4 tsp garlic powder

- 1/4 tsp paprika

- 1/4 tsp dried dill

- Salt and pepper to taste

- Lemon wedges for serving

Instructions:

1. Preheat the air fryer to 375°F.

2. Brush the salmon fillets with olive oil (optional) and season with garlic powder, paprika, dill, salt, and pepper.

3. Place the salmon fillets in the air fryer basket and cook for 8-10 minutes, depending on thickness, until flaky and cooked through.

4. Serve with a side of steamed vegetables or salad and a squeeze of fresh lemon.

4. Air-Fried Chicken and Veggie Skewers

Ingredients:

- 1 lb chicken breast, cut into cubes

- 1 bell pepper, cut into chunks

- 1 zucchini, sliced into rounds

- 1/2 red onion, cut into chunks

- 1/4 tsp garlic powder

- 1/4 tsp paprika

- 1/4 tsp oregano

- Salt and pepper to taste

Instructions:

1. Preheat the air fryer to 375°F.

2. In a bowl, toss the chicken cubes with garlic powder, paprika, oregano, salt, and pepper.

3. Thread the chicken and vegetables onto skewers.

4. Place the skewers in the air fryer basket and cook for 12-15 minutes, turning halfway through, until the chicken is cooked through.

5. Serve with a side of zero-point dipping sauce or a fresh salad.

5. Air-Fried Eggplant Lasagna Stacks

Ingredients:

- 1 medium eggplant, sliced into rounds

- 1/2 cup marinara sauce (sugar-free)

- 1/4 cup ricotta cheese (optional for low-point adaptation)

- 1/4 tsp Italian seasoning

- Salt and pepper to taste

- Fresh basil for garnish

Instructions:

1. Preheat the air fryer to 375°F.

2. Season the eggplant slices with salt and pepper. Air fry for 8-10 minutes, flipping halfway through, until tender.

3. On a plate, layer the eggplant slices with marinara sauce and ricotta cheese (if using). Repeat the layers to create a stack.

4. Return the stack to the air fryer for 2-3 minutes to heat through.

5. Garnish with fresh basil and serve as a delicious and hearty zero-point dinner.

6. Air-Fried Cajun Tilapia with Veggie Medley

Ingredients:

- 2 tilapia fillets

- 1/2 tsp Cajun seasoning

- 1/4 tsp garlic powder

- Salt and pepper to taste

- 1 cup broccoli florets

- 1/2 cup cherry tomatoes

- 1/2 cup zucchini, diced

Instructions:

1. Preheat the air fryer to 375°F.

2. Rub the tilapia fillets with Cajun seasoning, garlic powder, salt, and pepper.

3. Toss the veggies with a pinch of salt and pepper.

4. Place the tilapia and veggies in the air fryer basket and cook for 8-10 minutes, shaking the veggies halfway through.

5. Serve as a balanced, flavorful dinner.

7. Air-Fried Stuffed Bell Peppers

Ingredients:

- 2 large bell peppers, halved and seeded

- 1/2 cup cooked quinoa or cauliflower rice

- 1/4 cup black beans

- 1/4 cup diced tomatoes

- 1/4 tsp chili powder

- 1/4 tsp cumin

- Salt and pepper to taste

Instructions:

1. Preheat the air fryer to 375°F.

2. In a bowl, mix quinoa (or cauliflower rice), black beans, diced tomatoes, chili powder, cumin, salt, and pepper.

3. Stuff the bell pepper halves with the mixture.

4. Air fry the stuffed peppers for 10-12 minutes until the peppers are tender and the filling is heated through.

5. Garnish with fresh cilantro and enjoy!

8. Air-Fried Garlic Herb Chicken Thighs

Ingredients:

- 2 skinless, boneless chicken thighs

- 1/2 tsp garlic powder

- 1/4 tsp dried thyme

- 1/4 tsp paprika

- Salt and pepper to taste

Instructions:

1. Preheat the air fryer to 375°F.

2. Rub the chicken thighs with garlic powder, thyme, paprika, salt, and pepper.

3. Place the thighs in the air fryer and cook for 12-15 minutes, flipping halfway through, until cooked through and golden brown.

4. Serve with a side of steamed green beans or air-fried sweet potato wedges.

9. Air-Fried Ratatouille

Ingredients:

- 1/2 eggplant, diced

- 1 zucchini, diced

- 1 bell pepper, diced

- 1/4 cup onion, diced

- 1/2 cup diced tomatoes

- 1/4 tsp garlic powder

- 1/4 tsp dried basil

- Salt and pepper to taste

Instructions:

1. Preheat the air fryer to 375°F.

2. Toss all the vegetables with garlic powder, basil, salt, and pepper.

3. Air fry the vegetables for 10-12 minutes, shaking the basket halfway through, until tender.

4. Serve as a delicious vegetarian dinner or pair it with grilled protein for a heartier meal.

10. Air-Fried Lemon Herb Cod

Ingredients:

- 2 cod fillets

- 1 lemon, sliced

- 1/4 tsp garlic powder

- 1/4 tsp dried parsley

- Salt and pepper to taste

Instructions:

1. Preheat the air fryer to 375°F.

2. Season the cod fillets with garlic powder, parsley, salt, and pepper.

3. Place the fillets in the air fryer basket and top each with a lemon slice.

4. Air fry for 8-10 minutes, depending on the thickness of the fillets, until flaky and cooked through.

5. Serve with a side of steamed asparagus or air-fried Brussels sprouts.

11. Air-Fried Greek Chicken with Veggies

Ingredients:

- 2 skinless, boneless chicken breasts

- 1/2 cup cherry tomatoes

- 1/2 cup zucchini, diced

- 1/4 red onion, sliced

- 1/4 tsp garlic powder

- 1/4 tsp dried oregano

- Salt and pepper to taste

Instructions:

1. Preheat the air fryer to 375°F.

2. Season the chicken breasts with garlic powder, oregano, salt, and pepper.

3. Place the chicken and veggies in the air fryer basket.

4. Cook for 12-15 minutes, flipping the chicken and shaking the veggies halfway through, until the chicken is cooked through.

5. Serve with a sprinkle of fresh parsley or a lemon wedge for added flavor.

12. Air-Fried Cabbage Steaks

Ingredients:

- 1 small green cabbage, cut into 1-inch-thick slices

- 1/4 tsp garlic powder

- 1/4 tsp smoked paprika

- Salt and pepper to taste

- Optional: a squeeze of fresh lemon juice

Instructions:

1. Preheat the air fryer to 375°F.

2. Season the cabbage steaks with garlic powder, paprika, salt, and pepper.

3. Place the steaks in the air fryer basket and cook for 10-12 minutes, flipping halfway through, until tender and crispy on the edges.

4. Serve as a hearty vegetarian dinner or a side dish to your favorite protein.

13. Air-Fried Spaghetti Squash with Tomato Basil Sauce

Ingredients:

- 1 small spaghetti squash, halved and seeded

- 1/2 cup sugar-free marinara sauce

- 1/4 tsp garlic powder

- Fresh basil for garnish

Instructions:

1. Preheat the air fryer to 375°F.

2. Place the spaghetti squash halves, cut side down, in the air fryer basket. Cook for 15-20 minutes, depending on size, until tender.

3. Scrape the flesh with a fork to create spaghetti-like strands.

4. Heat the marinara sauce and serve it over the squash. Garnish with fresh basil for a light and satisfying dinner.

14. Air-Fried Asian-Inspired Salmon

Ingredients:

- 2 salmon fillets

- 1 tsp low-sodium soy sauce

- 1/2 tsp grated ginger

- 1 garlic clove, minced

- 1/2 tsp sesame seeds (optional)

Instructions:

1. Preheat the air fryer to 375°F.

2. In a small bowl, mix soy sauce, ginger, and garlic. Brush the mixture over the salmon fillets.

3. Place the salmon in the air fryer basket and cook for 8-10 minutes, until the salmon is flaky and cooked through.

4. Sprinkle with sesame seeds (if using) and serve with a side of steamed broccoli or snap peas.

15. Air-Fried Portobello Mushroom Burgers

Ingredients:

- 2 large portobello mushroom caps

- 1/4 tsp garlic powder

- 1/4 tsp smoked paprika

- 1/4 tsp dried thyme

- Salt and pepper to taste

- Lettuce leaves and sliced tomato for serving

Instructions:

1. Preheat the air fryer to 375°F.

2. Season the mushroom caps with garlic powder, paprika, thyme, salt, and pepper.

3. Place the mushrooms in the air fryer basket and cook for 8-10 minutes, flipping halfway through, until tender.

4. Serve on lettuce leaves with sliced tomato and your favorite zero-point condiments for a hearty and healthy burger alternative.

These Zero Point Air Fryer Dinner Recipes offer a variety of tastes and textures to suit every craving.

From hearty mushroom burgers to light spaghetti squash, there's something for everyone to enjoy while staying on track!

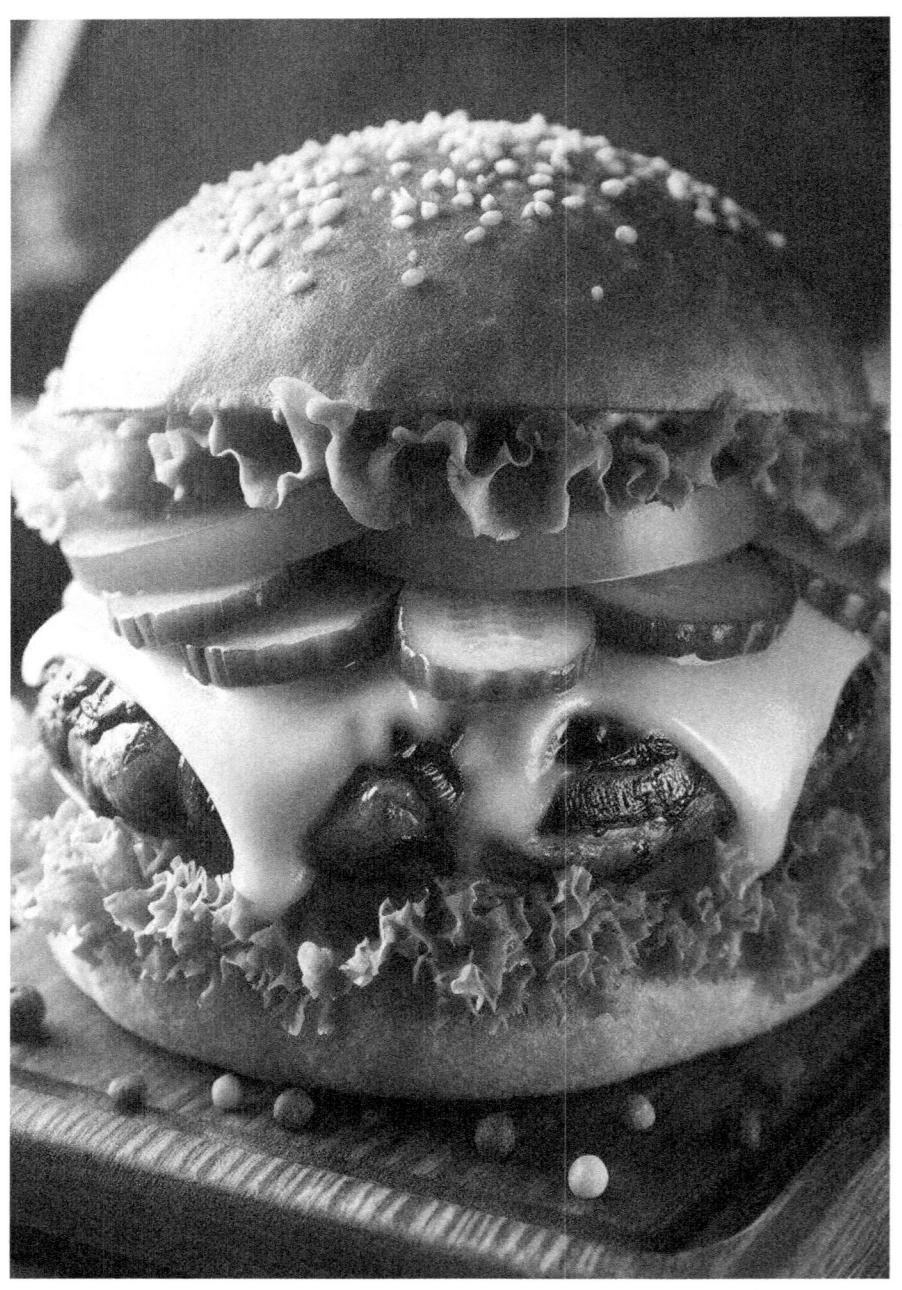

CHAPTER FIVE

Zero Point Air Fryer Snacks

1. Air-Fried Zucchini Chips

Ingredients:

- 1 medium zucchini, thinly sliced

- 1/4 tsp garlic powder

- 1/4 tsp smoked paprika

- Salt and pepper to taste

Instructions:

1. Preheat the air fryer to 375°F.

2. Pat the zucchini slices dry with a paper towel and season with garlic powder, paprika, salt, and pepper.

3. Place the slices in a single layer in the air fryer basket.

4. Air fry for 8-10 minutes, flipping halfway through, until crispy.

5. Serve as a crunchy snack or dip into a zero-point salsa.

2. Air-Fried Spiced Chickpeas

Ingredients:

- 1 cup canned chickpeas, drained and rinsed

- 1/4 tsp cumin

- 1/4 tsp chili powder

- 1/4 tsp garlic powder

- Salt to taste

Instructions:

1. Preheat the air fryer to 400°F.

2. Pat the chickpeas dry with a paper towel and toss with spices and salt.

3. Spread the chickpeas in the air fryer basket in a single layer.

4. Air fry for 10-12 minutes, shaking the basket halfway through, until golden and crunchy.

5. Cool slightly before enjoying as a high-protein snack.

3. Air-Fried Apple Slices with Cinnamon

Ingredients:

- 1 apple, thinly sliced

- 1/4 tsp cinnamon

Instructions:

1. Preheat the air fryer to 375°F.

2. Toss the apple slices with cinnamon.

3. Arrange the slices in the air fryer basket in a single layer.

4. Air fry for 6-8 minutes, flipping halfway through, until tender and slightly caramelized.

5. Enjoy as a naturally sweet and healthy snack.

4. Air-Fried Buffalo Cauliflower Bites

Ingredients:

- 2 cups cauliflower florets

- 1/4 cup hot sauce (zero-point)

- 1/4 tsp garlic powder

Instructions:

1. Preheat the air fryer to 375°F.

2. Toss the cauliflower florets with hot sauce and garlic powder.

3. Spread the florets in the air fryer basket in a single layer.

4. Air fry for 10-12 minutes, shaking halfway through, until the florets are crispy and lightly browned.

5. Serve with celery sticks for a classic pairing.

5. Air-Fried Eggplant Fries

Ingredients:

- 1 small eggplant, cut into fry-shaped sticks

- 1/4 tsp garlic powder

- 1/4 tsp Italian seasoning

- Salt to taste

Instructions:

1. Preheat the air fryer to 375°F.

2. Toss the eggplant sticks with garlic powder, Italian seasoning, and salt.

3. Place the sticks in the air fryer basket in a single layer.

4. Air fry for 10-12 minutes, flipping halfway through, until golden and tender.

5. Serve with a zero-point marinara sauce for dipping.

6. Air-Fried Kale Chips

Ingredients:

- 2 cups kale leaves, stems removed and torn into bite-sized pieces

- 1/4 tsp garlic powder

- 1/4 tsp smoked paprika

- Salt to taste

Instructions:

1. Preheat the air fryer to 375°F.

2. Massage the kale leaves with garlic powder, paprika, and a pinch of salt.

3. Spread the leaves in a single layer in the air fryer basket.

4. Air fry for 4-6 minutes, shaking the basket halfway through, until crispy.

5. Enjoy these crunchy chips as a savory snack!

7. Air-Fried Bell Pepper Nachos

Ingredients:

- 1 large bell pepper, sliced into wide strips

- 1/4 cup black beans

- 1/4 cup diced tomatoes

- 1/4 tsp chili powder

- Optional: fresh cilantro for garnish

Instructions:

1. Preheat the air fryer to 375°F.

2. Arrange the bell pepper slices in the air fryer basket. Air fry for 5 minutes until slightly tender.

3. Top with black beans, diced tomatoes, and a sprinkle of chili powder. Air fry for an additional 2-3 minutes.

4. Garnish with fresh cilantro and enjoy as a fun, zero-point nacho alternative!

8. Air-Fried Carrot Fries

Ingredients:

- 2 large carrots, peeled and cut into fry shapes

- 1/4 tsp garlic powder

- 1/4 tsp cumin

- Salt and pepper to taste

Instructions:

1. Preheat the air fryer to 375°F.

2. Toss the carrot fries with garlic powder, cumin, salt, and pepper.

3. Spread the fries in the air fryer basket in a single layer.

4. Air fry for 10-12 minutes, shaking halfway through, until tender and slightly crispy on the edges.

5. Serve with a zero-point dip or enjoy as-is.

9. Air-Fried Edamame

Ingredients:

- 1 cup shelled edamame (frozen or fresh)

- 1/4 tsp garlic powder

- 1/4 tsp chili flakes (optional)

- Salt to taste

Instructions:

1. Preheat the air fryer to 375°F.

2. Toss the edamame with garlic powder, chili flakes (if using), and a pinch of salt.

3. Spread in the air fryer basket in a single layer.

4. Air fry for 8-10 minutes, shaking halfway through, until the edges are slightly crispy.

5. Serve warm as a protein-packed snack.

10. Air-Fried Radish Chips

Ingredients:

- 1 cup radishes, thinly sliced

- 1/4 tsp garlic powder

- 1/4 tsp dried dill

- Salt to taste

Instructions:

1. Preheat the air fryer to 375°F.

2. Toss the radish slices with garlic powder, dried dill, and a pinch of salt.

3. Arrange the slices in the air fryer basket in a single layer.

4. Air fry for 8-10 minutes, shaking halfway through, until crispy.

5. Enjoy this low-carb, crunchy snack anytime!

CHAPTER SIX

Zero Point Air Fryer Dessert

1. Air-Fried Cinnamon Apples

Ingredients:

- 1 apple, sliced into thin wedges

- 1/2 tsp ground cinnamon

Instructions:

1. Preheat the air fryer to 375°F.

2. Toss the apple slices with cinnamon.

3. Arrange the slices in a single layer in the air fryer basket.

4. Air fry for 8-10 minutes, shaking halfway through, until tender and lightly caramelized.

5. Serve warm as a naturally sweet dessert.

2. Air-Fried Banana Slices with Cocoa Dusting

Ingredients:

- 1 ripe banana, sliced

- 1/4 tsp unsweetened cocoa powder

Instructions:

1. Preheat the air fryer to 350°F.

2. Arrange the banana slices in a single layer in the air fryer basket.

3. Air fry for 5-6 minutes until golden and slightly crispy on the edges.

4. Sprinkle with unsweetened cocoa powder before serving.

3. Air-Fried Pineapple Rings

Ingredients:

- 4 fresh pineapple rings

- 1/4 tsp ground cinnamon

Instructions:

1. Preheat the air fryer to 375°F.

2. Sprinkle cinnamon on both sides of the pineapple rings.

3. Place the rings in the air fryer basket in a single layer.

4. Air fry for 8-10 minutes, flipping halfway through, until the pineapple is warm and caramelized.

5. Serve as-is or with a dollop of zero-point whipped topping.

4. Air-Fried Pear Halves with Nutmeg

Ingredients:

- 1 ripe pear, halved and cored

- 1/4 tsp ground nutmeg

Instructions:

1. Preheat the air fryer to 375°F.

2. Sprinkle the pear halves with nutmeg.

3. Place the pears in the air fryer basket, cut side up.

4. Air fry for 10-12 minutes until the pears are tender and lightly browned.

5. Enjoy warm for a simple, elegant dessert.

5. Air-Fried Peaches with Cinnamon and Vanilla

Ingredients:

- 2 ripe peaches, halved and pitted

- 1/2 tsp ground cinnamon

- 1/2 tsp vanilla extract

Instructions:

1. Preheat the air fryer to 375°F.

2. Brush the peach halves with vanilla extract and sprinkle with cinnamon.

3. Place the peaches in the air fryer basket, cut side up.

4. Air fry for 8-10 minutes until tender and caramelized.

5. Serve warm as a delightful zero-point dessert.

6. Air-Fried Grapefruit with Cinnamon Sugar Alternative

Ingredients:

- 1 large grapefruit, halved

- 1/4 tsp cinnamon

- A sprinkle of a zero-calorie sweetener (optional)

Instructions:

1. Preheat the air fryer to 375°F.

2. Sprinkle the cut side of the grapefruit halves with cinnamon and a zero-calorie sweetener.

3. Place the grapefruit halves in the air fryer basket, cut side up.

4. Air fry for 6-8 minutes until the top is lightly caramelized.

5. Serve warm for a zesty, sweet treat.

7. Air-Fried Mango Slices

Ingredients:

- 1 ripe mango, peeled and sliced into strips

- 1/4 tsp chili powder (optional, for a spicy twist)

Instructions:

1. Preheat the air fryer to 375°F.

2. Toss the mango slices with chili powder for a sweet and spicy combo, or leave them plain.

3. Arrange the slices in the air fryer basket in a single layer.

4. Air fry for 6-8 minutes until warm and slightly caramelized.

5. Enjoy as a tropical, juicy dessert!

8. Air-Fried Mixed Berry Compote

Ingredients:

- 1 cup mixed berries (strawberries, blueberries, raspberries)

- 1/2 tsp vanilla extract

Instructions:

1. Preheat the air fryer to 350°F.

2. Toss the berries with vanilla extract and place them in a small oven-safe dish that fits in the air fryer.

3. Cook for 6-8 minutes until the berries soften and release their juices.

4. Serve warm over zero-point yogurt or enjoy as-is.

9. Air-Fried Stuffed Apples with Date Filling

Ingredients:

- 1 medium apple, cored

- 1 medjool date, finely chopped

- 1/4 tsp cinnamon

Instructions:

1. Preheat the air fryer to 375°F.

2. Mix the chopped date with cinnamon and stuff it into the cored apple.

3. Place the apple in the air fryer basket and cook for 12-15 minutes until soft and golden.

4. Let it cool slightly before serving for a naturally sweet dessert.

10. Air-Fried Strawberry "Shortcakes"

Ingredients:

- 1 cup fresh strawberries, halved

- Zero-point whipped topping or plain Greek yogurt for serving

Instructions:

1. Preheat the air fryer to 350°F.

2. Place the strawberries in a small oven-safe dish that fits in the air fryer.

3. Cook for 6-8 minutes until the strawberries are softened and their juices thicken.

4. Spoon the warm strawberries over whipped topping or yogurt for a light, zero-point dessert.

These Zero Point Air Fryer Dessert Recipes bring creativity and natural sweetness to your menu, offering indulgence without compromise!

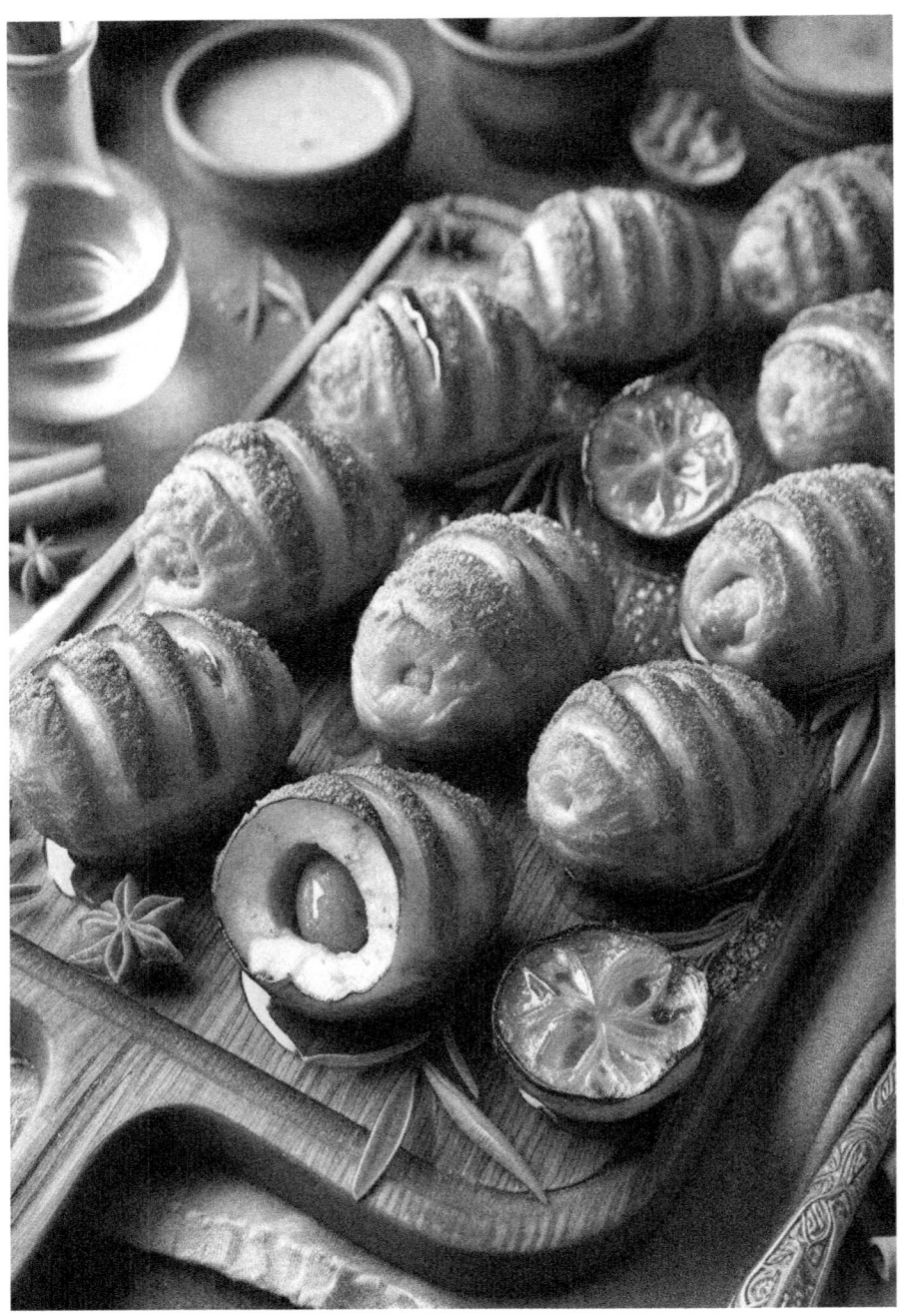

CONCLUSION

Congratulations on taking the first step toward a healthier, simpler, and more delicious way of living with The Zero Point Air Fryer Cookbook 2025! Throughout this book, we've explored the power of zero-point recipes, the convenience of air frying, and the joy of preparing meals that are as nutritious as they are satisfying.

Your air fryer is more than just a kitchen gadget; it's a gateway to effortless cooking and smart choices. By embracing the principles of zero-point eating, you've unlocked the ability to enjoy meals and snacks without the constant worry of counting calories or compromising flavor. The recipes and meal plans provided in this book are designed to inspire creativity, make mealtime exciting, and fit seamlessly into your busy lifestyle.

The journey toward weight loss and better health doesn't have to be about deprivation—it's about abundance: vibrant, wholesome ingredients, exciting flavors, and the freedom to enjoy food that supports your goals.

Whether you're enjoying a crispy breakfast, a hearty lunch, a satisfying dinner, or a guilt-free snack or dessert, every recipe in this book has been crafted to empower you on your journey.

As you continue to experiment with these recipes, remember that success isn't about perfection—it's about progress. Celebrate each step you take, every meal you prepare, and every healthy choice you make. Use this book as a guide, but don't hesitate to adapt recipes to suit your personal preferences or dietary needs.

What's Next?

The possibilities are endless! With your newfound knowledge of zero-point cooking and the versatility of your air fryer, you're equipped to create a lifestyle that's not just sustainable but also enjoyable. Share these recipes with family and friends, and inspire others to join you on this journey. Your choices today can have a ripple effect, helping others see that healthy eating can be simple, fun, and delicious.

A Final Thought

Thank you for choosing The Zero Point Air Fryer Cookbook 2025 as your companion on this journey. Remember, the key to lasting success is consistency, balance, and enjoying the process. Your air fryer is ready, the recipes are here, and the best version of yourself is waiting—one flavorful bite at a time.

Take Action Now

Ready to transform your kitchen and your life? Dive into these recipes, try the meal plans, and savor every moment of your health journey. Let this book be your motivation to continue making choices that nourish your body, fuel your spirit, and celebrate the joy of food.

Here's to a healthier, happier, and absolutely delicious future!

Printed in Great Britain
by Amazon